AF575670

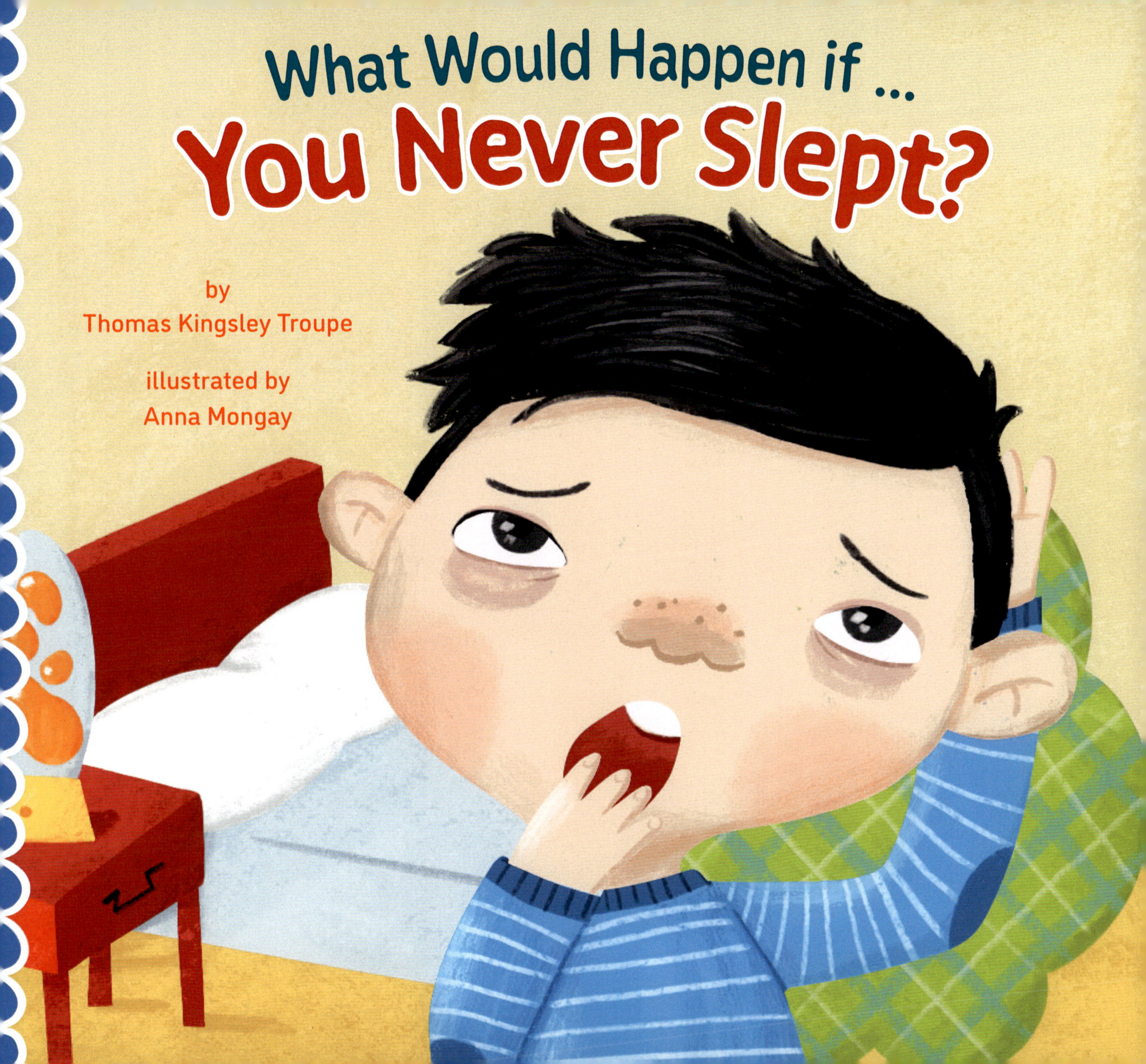

What Would Happen if ... You Never Slept?

by
Thomas Kingsley Troupe

illustrated by
Anna Mongay

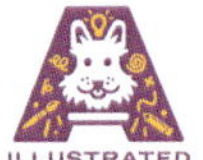

Published in 2024 by Amicus Learning, an imprint of Amicus
P.O. Box 227, Mankato MN 56002
www.amicuspublishing.us

Cataloging-in-Publication data is available from the Library of Congress.
Library Binding ISBN: 9781645492924
Paperback ISBN: 9781681528168
eBook ISBN: 9781645493808

LCCN: 2023011927

Editor: Rebecca Glaser
Designer: Lori Bye

ABOUT THE AUTHOR

Thomas Kingsley Troupe is the author of more than 200 books for children. When he's not writing, he likes to read, play video games, and recall when he last took a shower. Thomas is an expert nap-taker who lives in Woodbury, Minnesota, with his two sons.

ABOUT THE ILLUSTRATOR

Anna Mongay was born in Barcelona, Spain. As a child, she liked to draw, ride bikes, and run in the mountains. After studying fine arts and scenography at the University of Fine Arts in Barcelona, she now lives and works in Pacs del Penedès, Spain, as an illustrator and teacher.

Anna acknowledges the late Susana Hoslet, fellow illustrator, for her contributions to the art for this series.

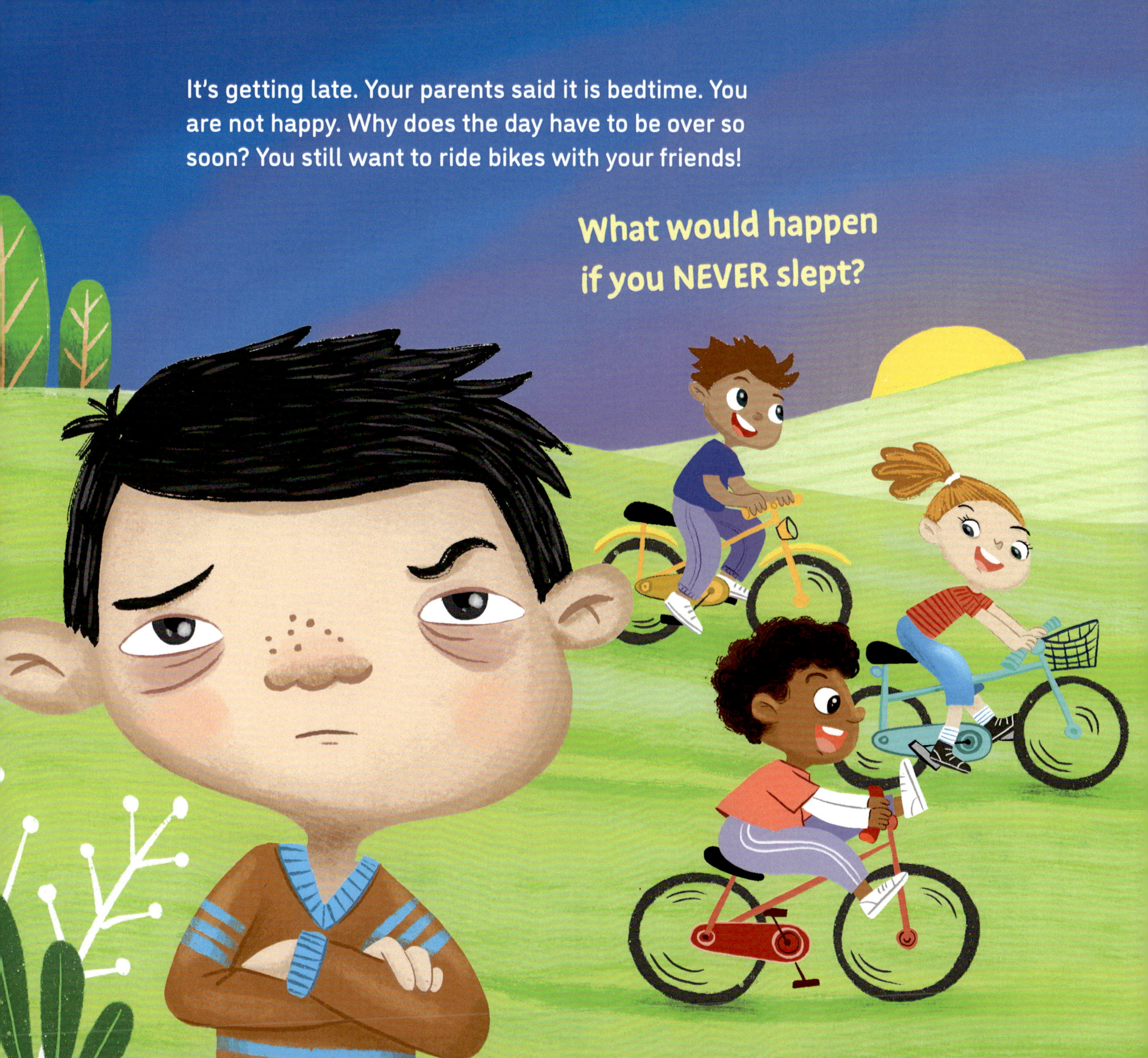

It's getting late. Your parents said it is bedtime. You are not happy. Why does the day have to be over so soon? You still want to ride bikes with your friends!

What would happen if you NEVER slept?

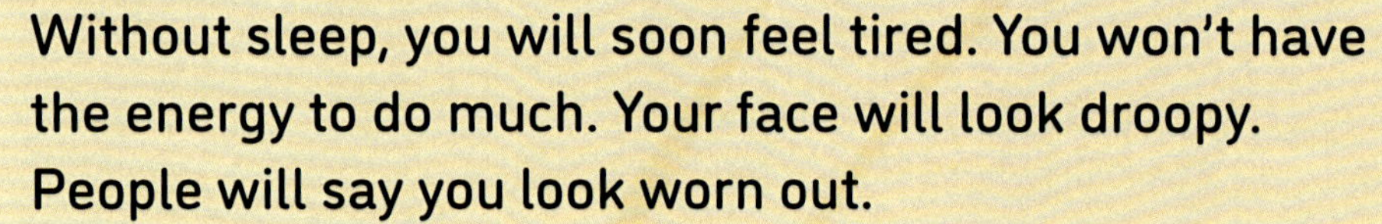

Without sleep, you will soon feel tired. You won't have the energy to do much. Your face will look droopy. People will say you look worn out.

You will feel like taking a nap. But then, your body might do something strange . . .

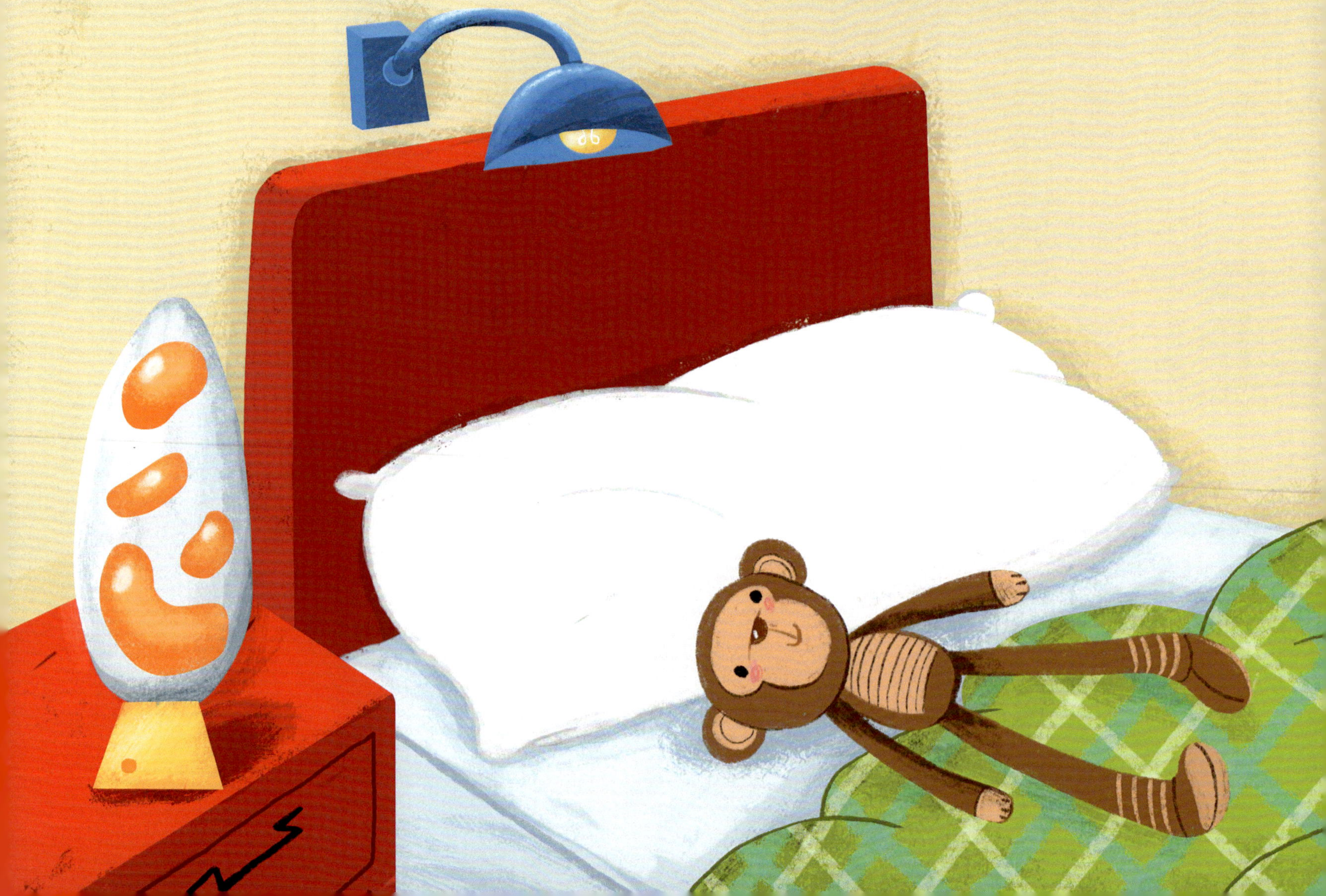

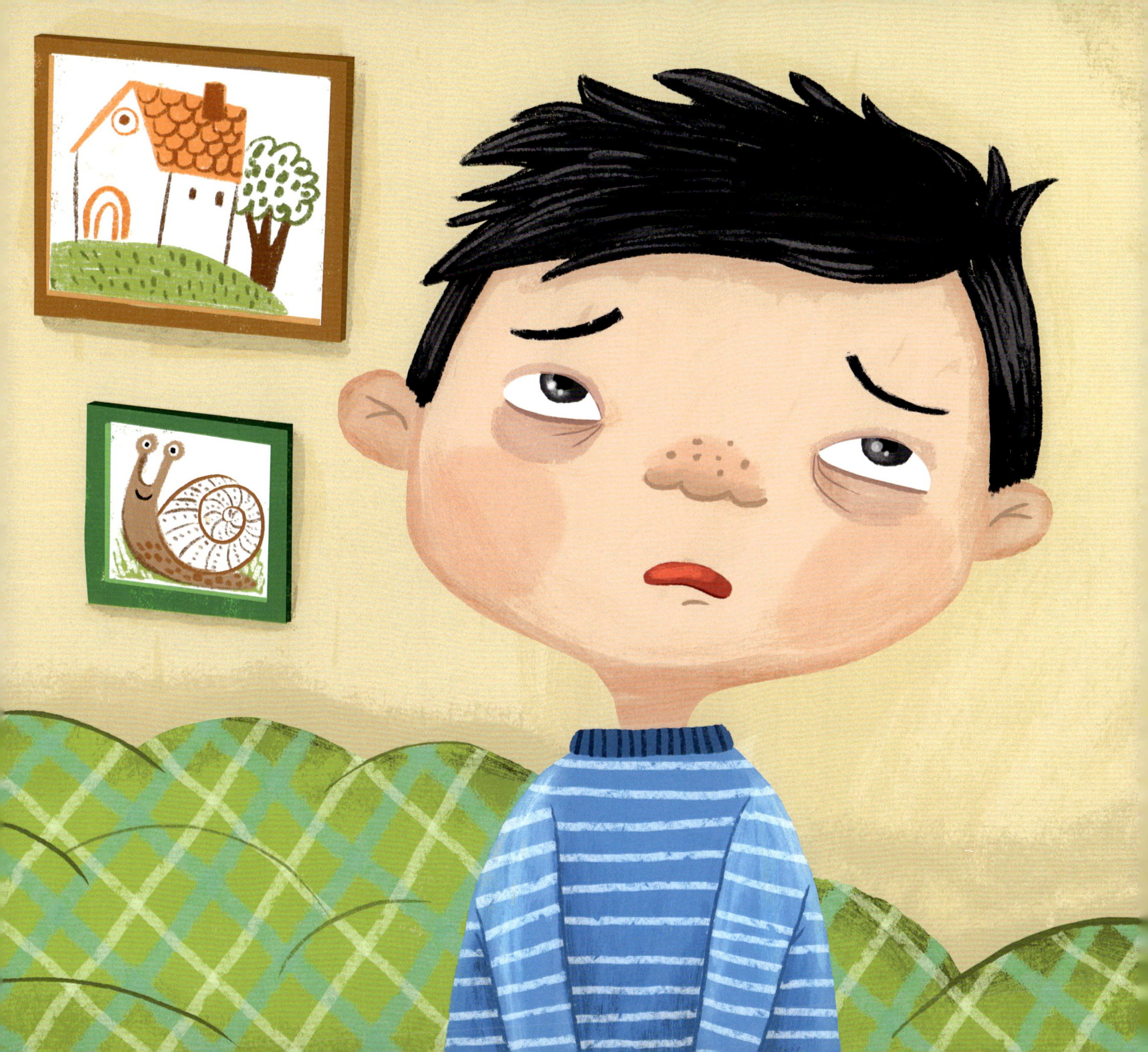

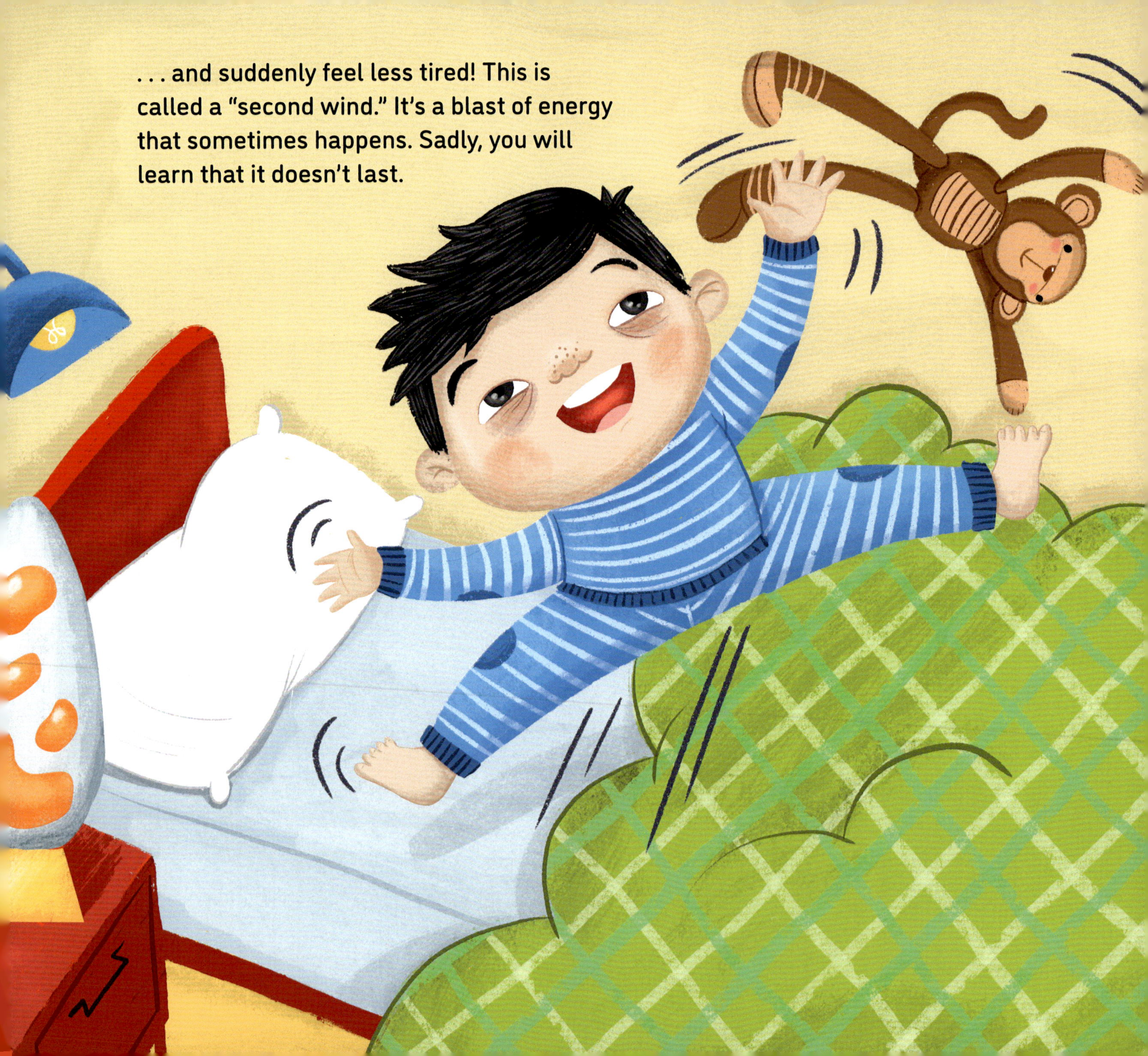

. . . and suddenly feel less tired! This is called a "second wind." It's a blast of energy that sometimes happens. Sadly, you will learn that it doesn't last.

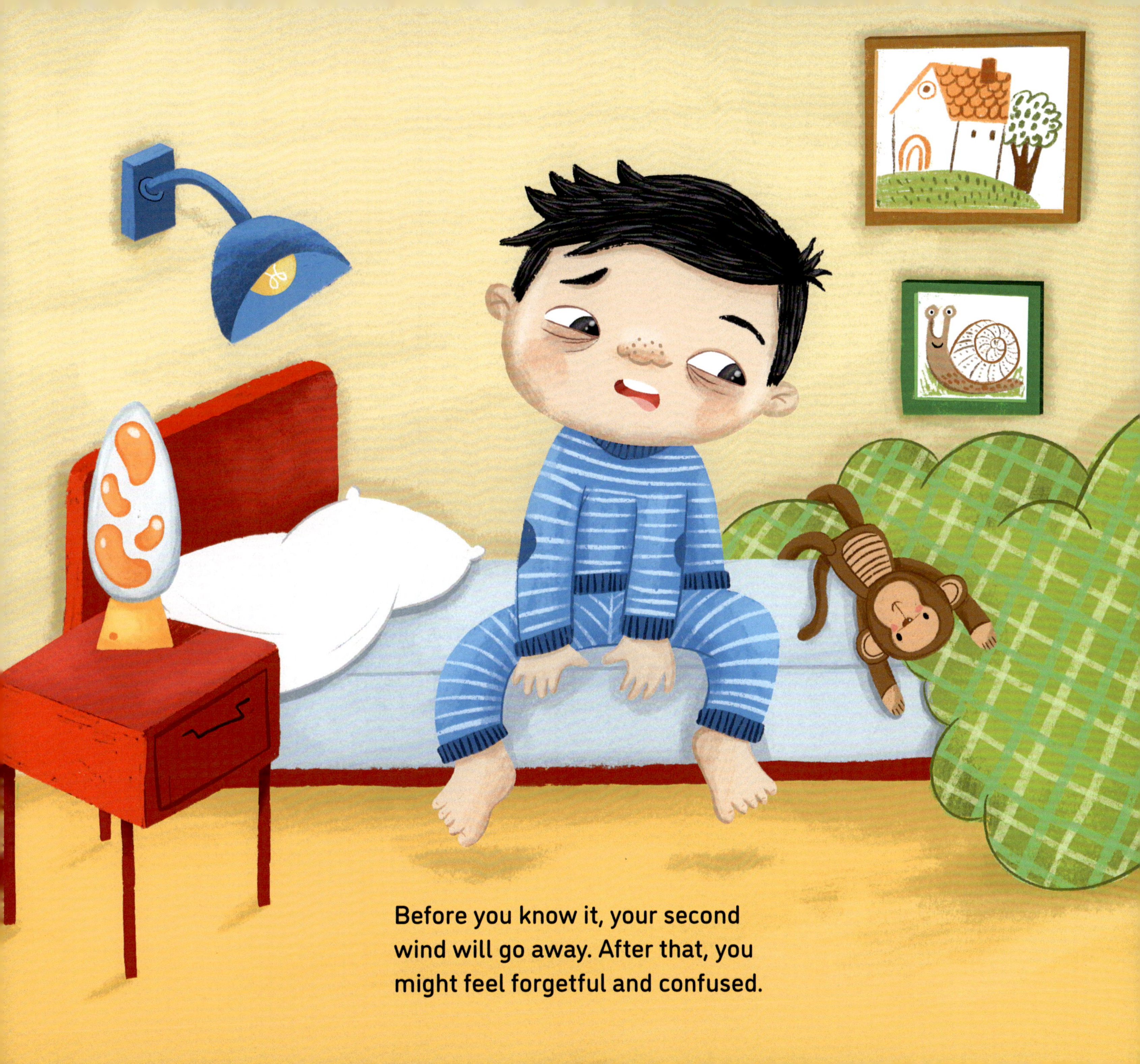

Before you know it, your second wind will go away. After that, you might feel forgetful and confused.

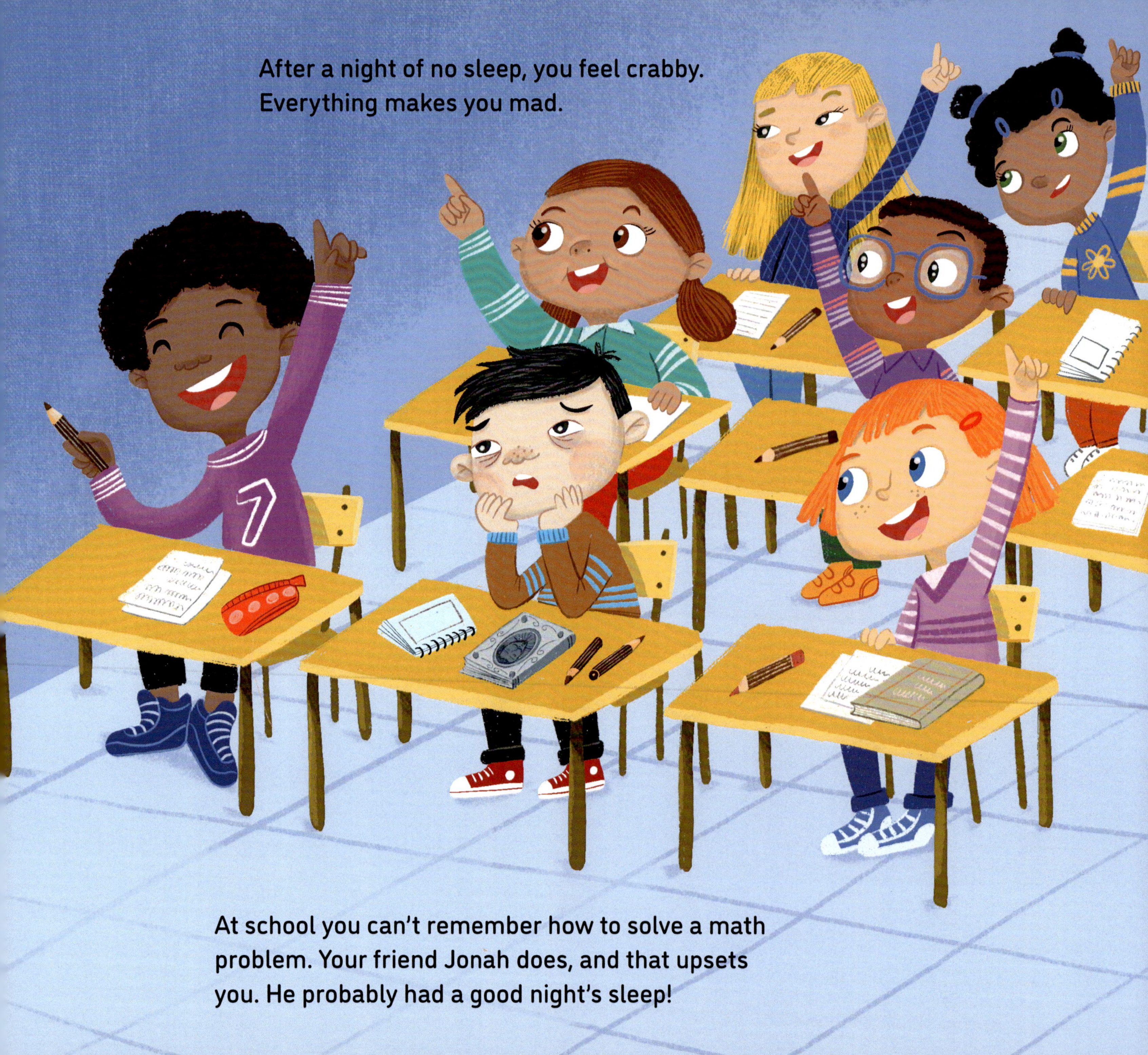

After a night of no sleep, you feel crabby. Everything makes you mad.

At school you can't remember how to solve a math problem. Your friend Jonah does, and that upsets you. He probably had a good night's sleep!

You're even angry at the smell of Ruby's sandwich!

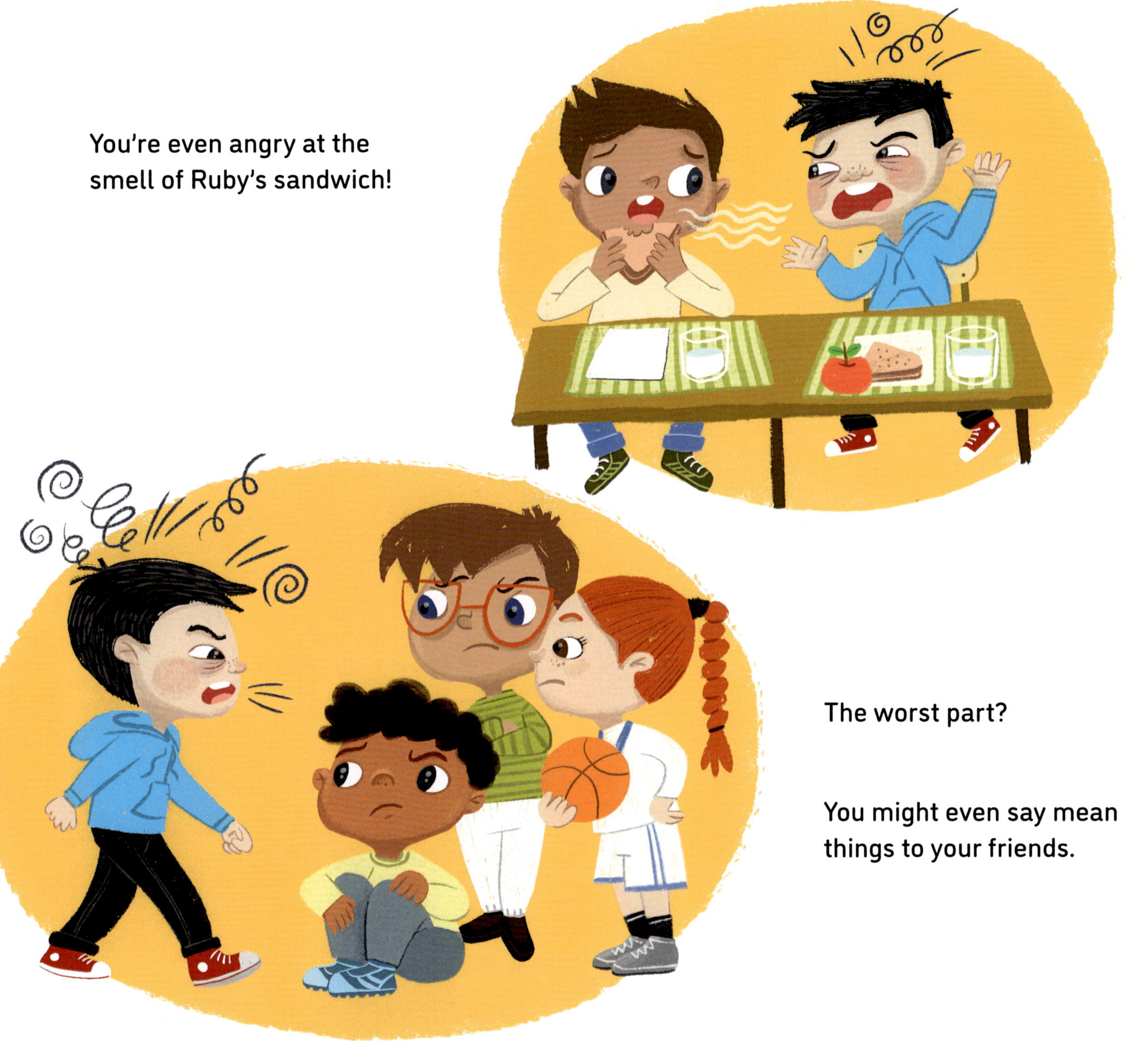

The worst part?

You might even say mean things to your friends.

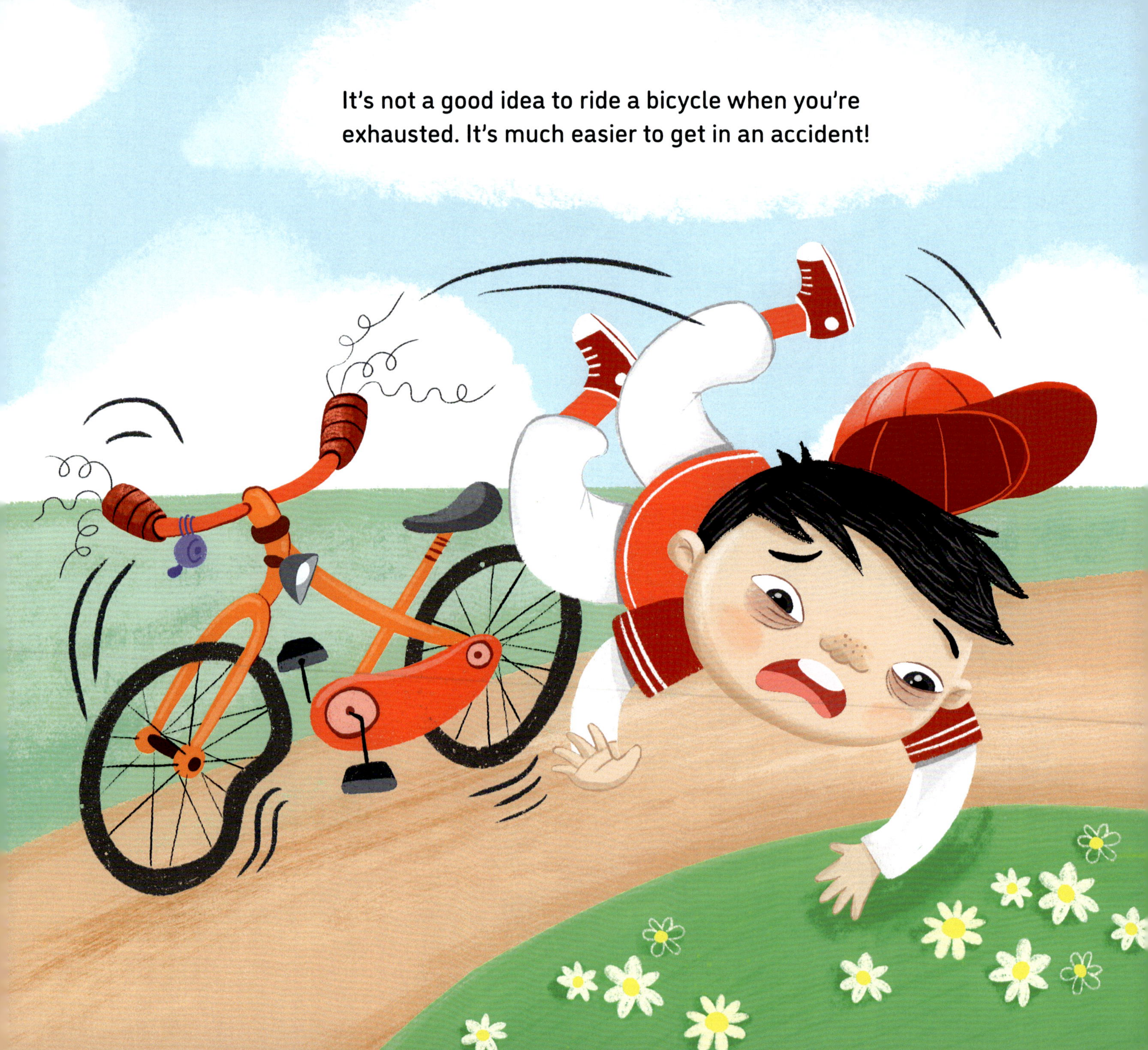

It’s not a good idea to ride a bicycle when you’re exhausted. It’s much easier to get in an accident!

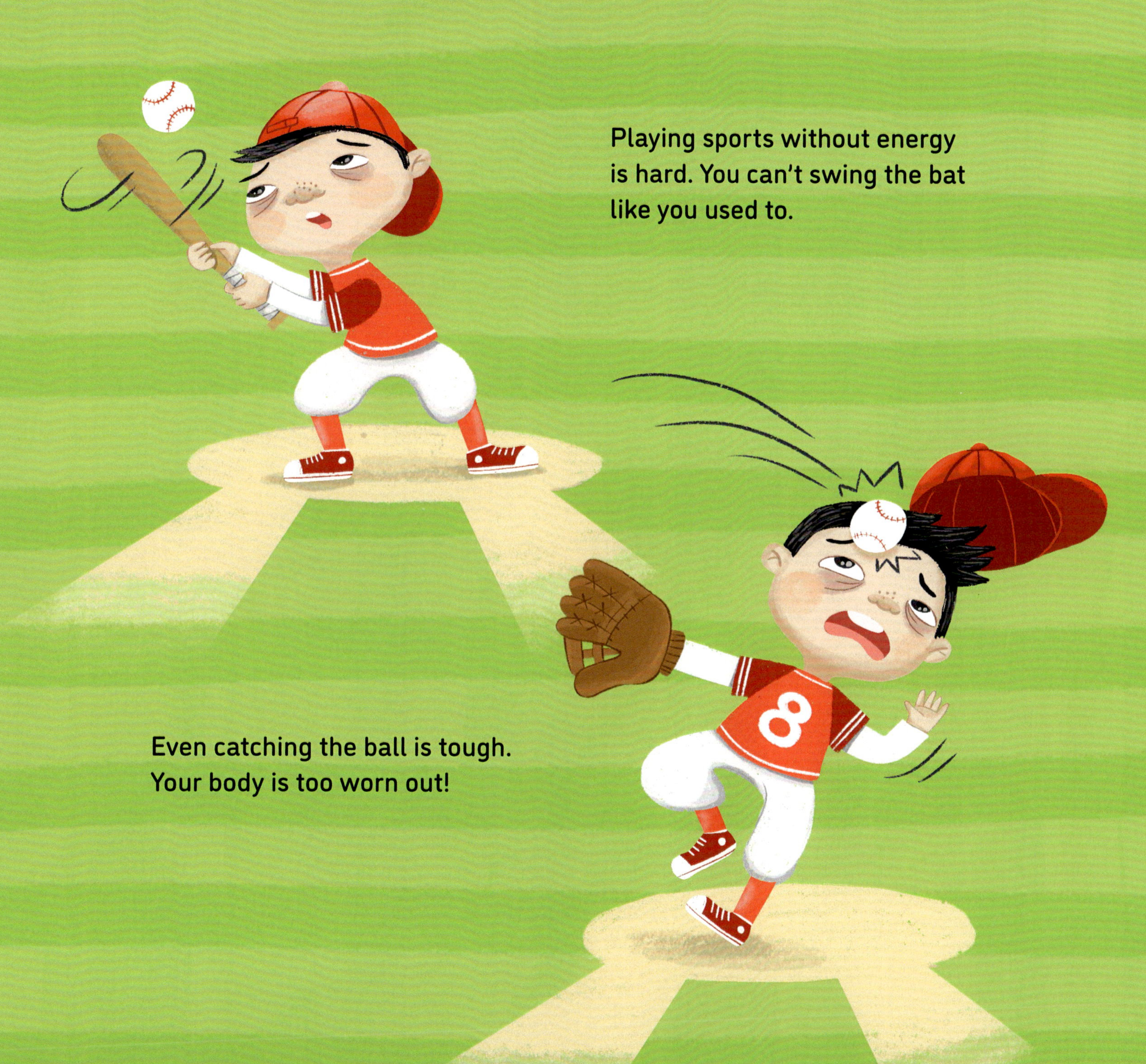

Playing sports without energy is hard. You can't swing the bat like you used to.

Even catching the ball is tough. Your body is too worn out!

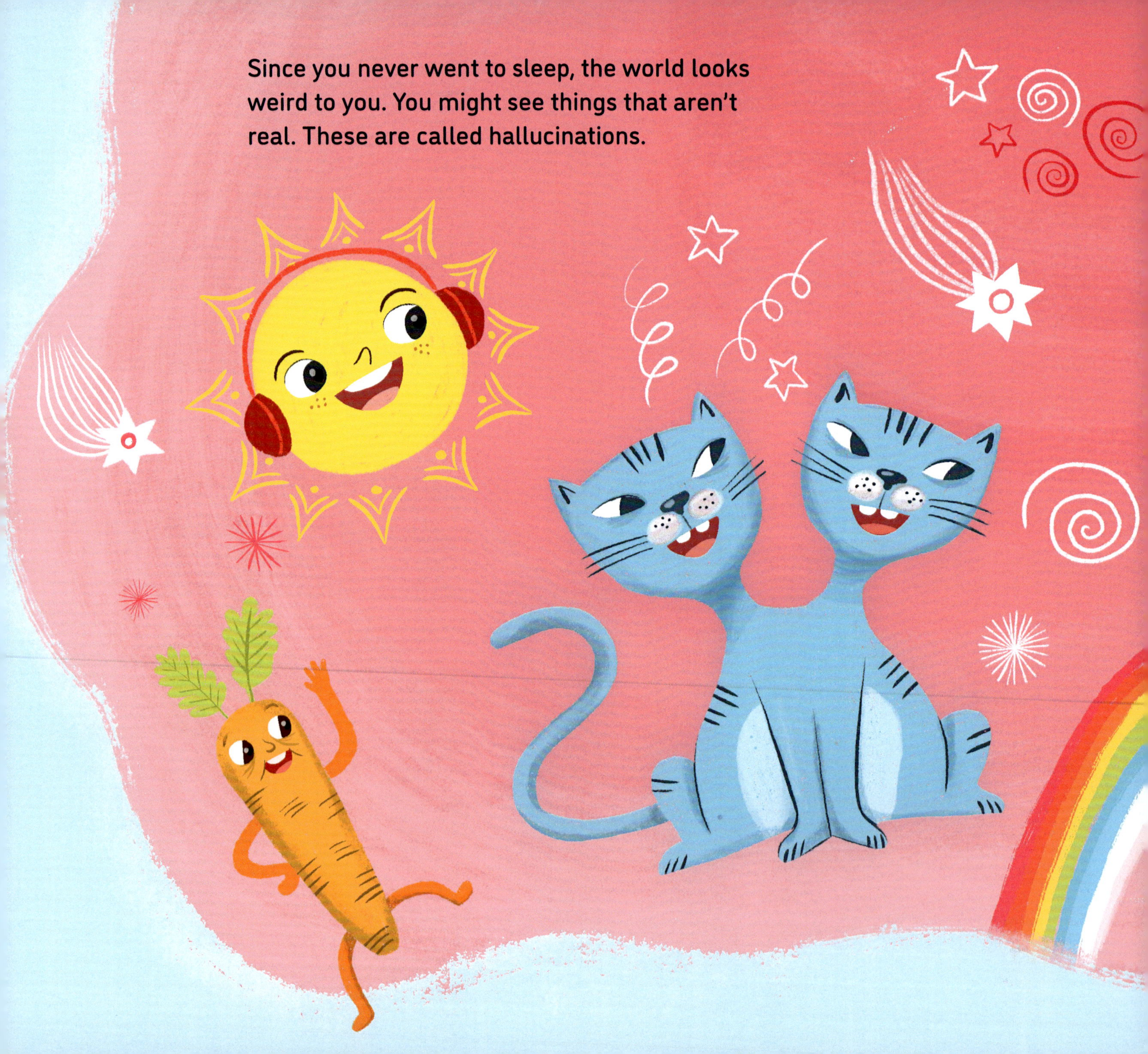

Since you never went to sleep, the world looks weird to you. You might see things that aren't real. These are called hallucinations.

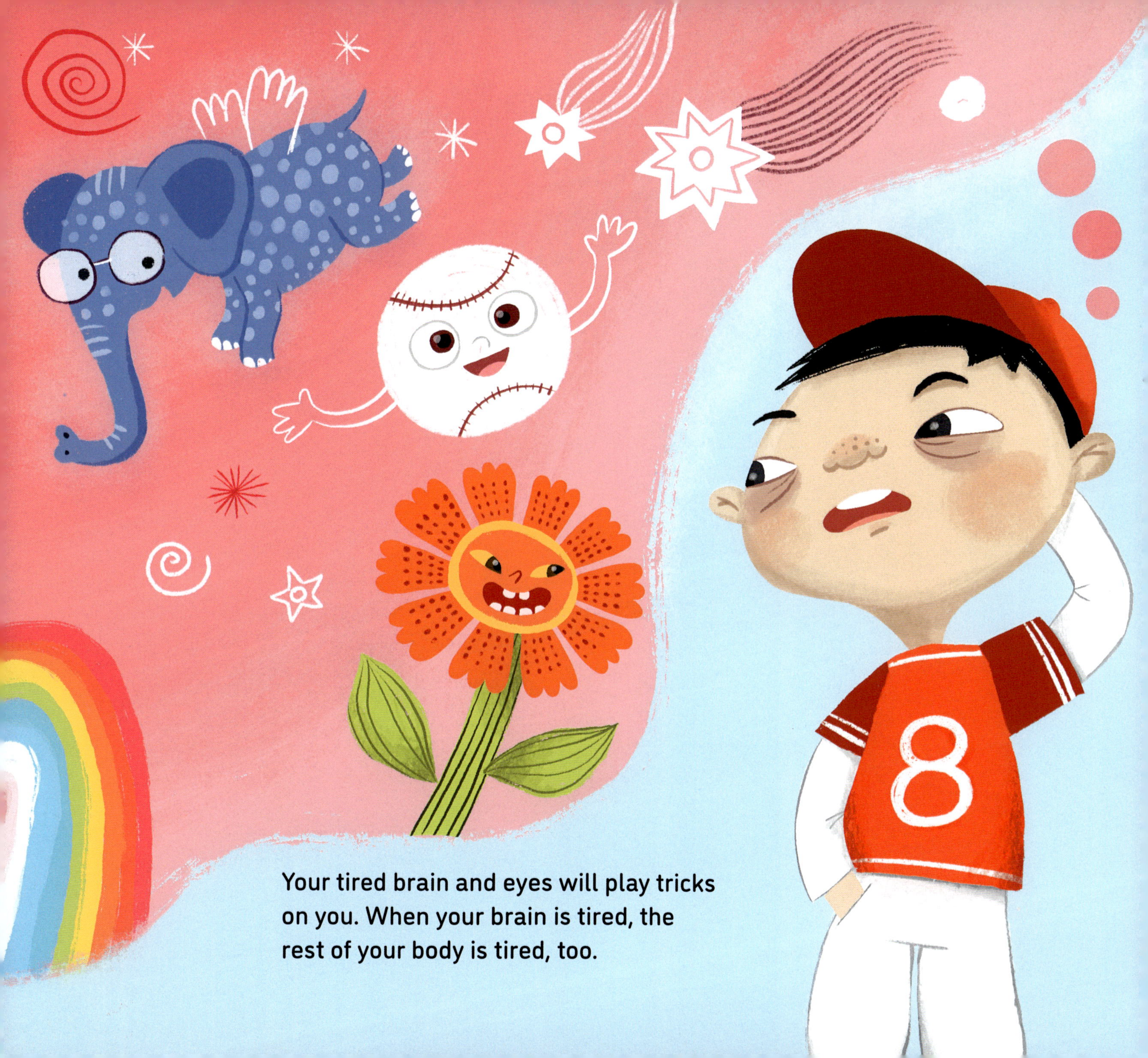

Your tired brain and eyes will play tricks on you. When your brain is tired, the rest of your body is tired, too.

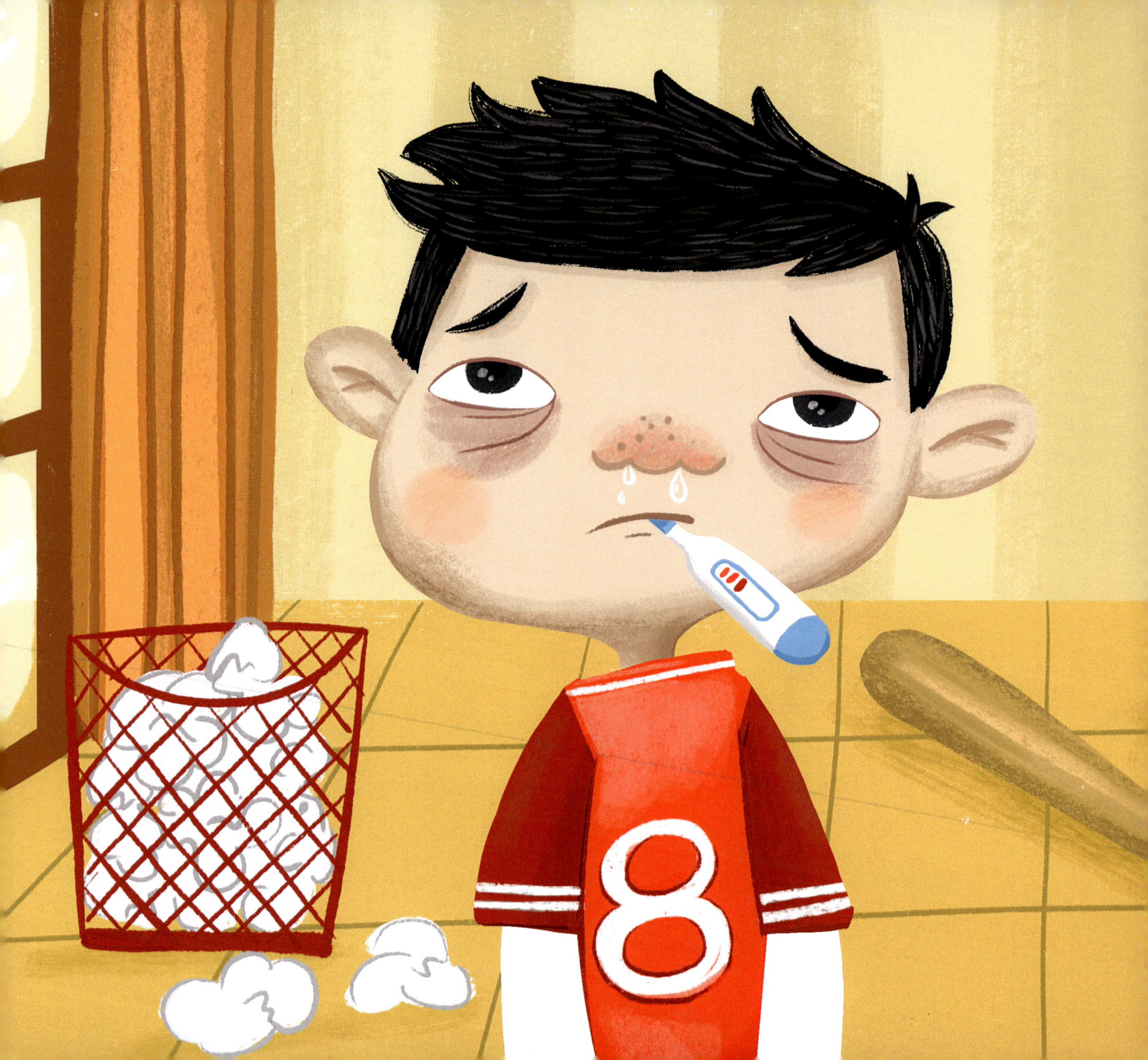
8

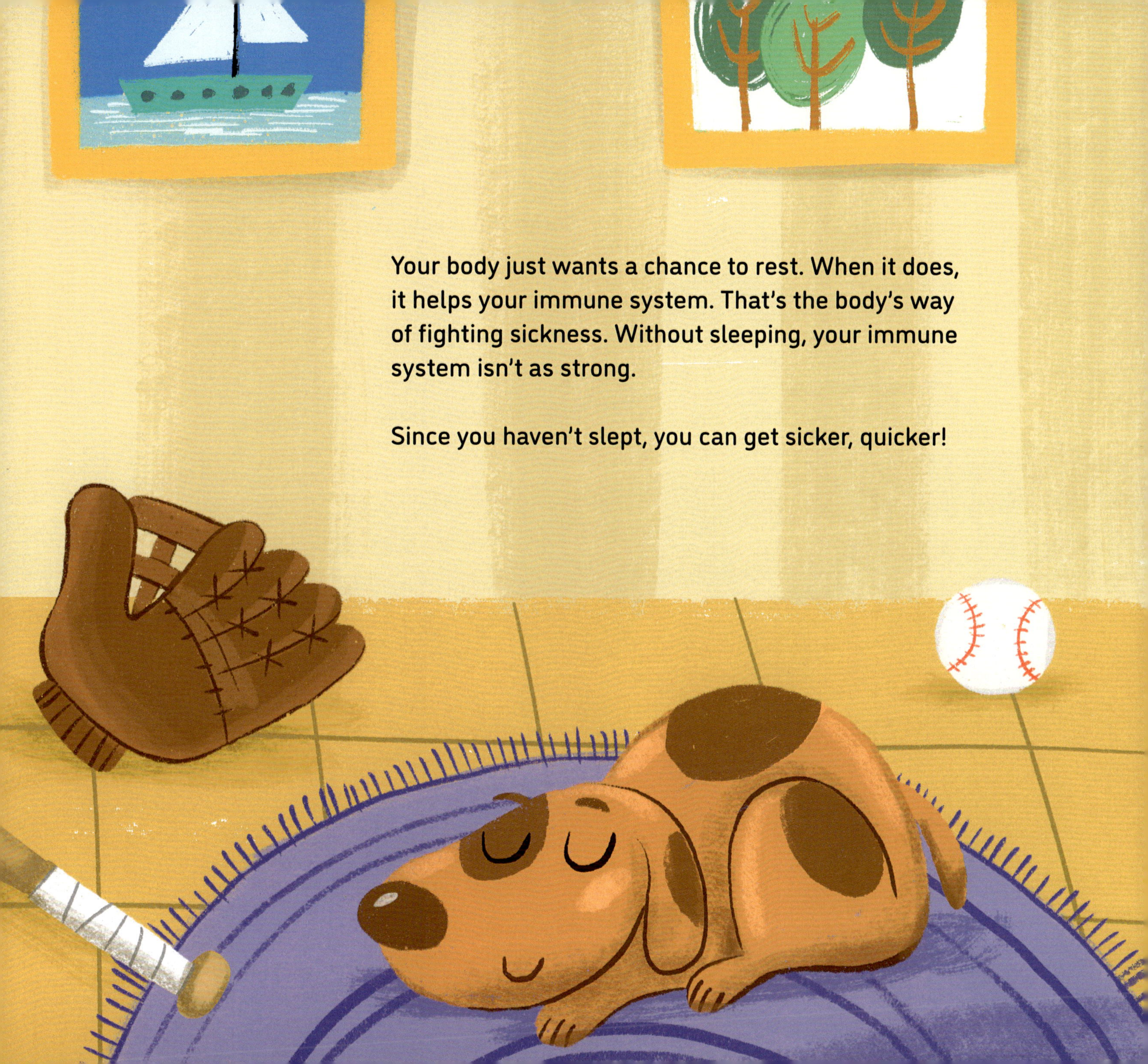

Your body just wants a chance to rest. When it does, it helps your immune system. That's the body's way of fighting sickness. Without sleeping, your immune system isn't as strong.

Since you haven't slept, you can get sicker, quicker!

Bed looks really good to you. Your body thinks you're making a good choice. You are giving your brain and body a chance to rest and repair.

Some sleep is better than no sleep. More sleep is even better!

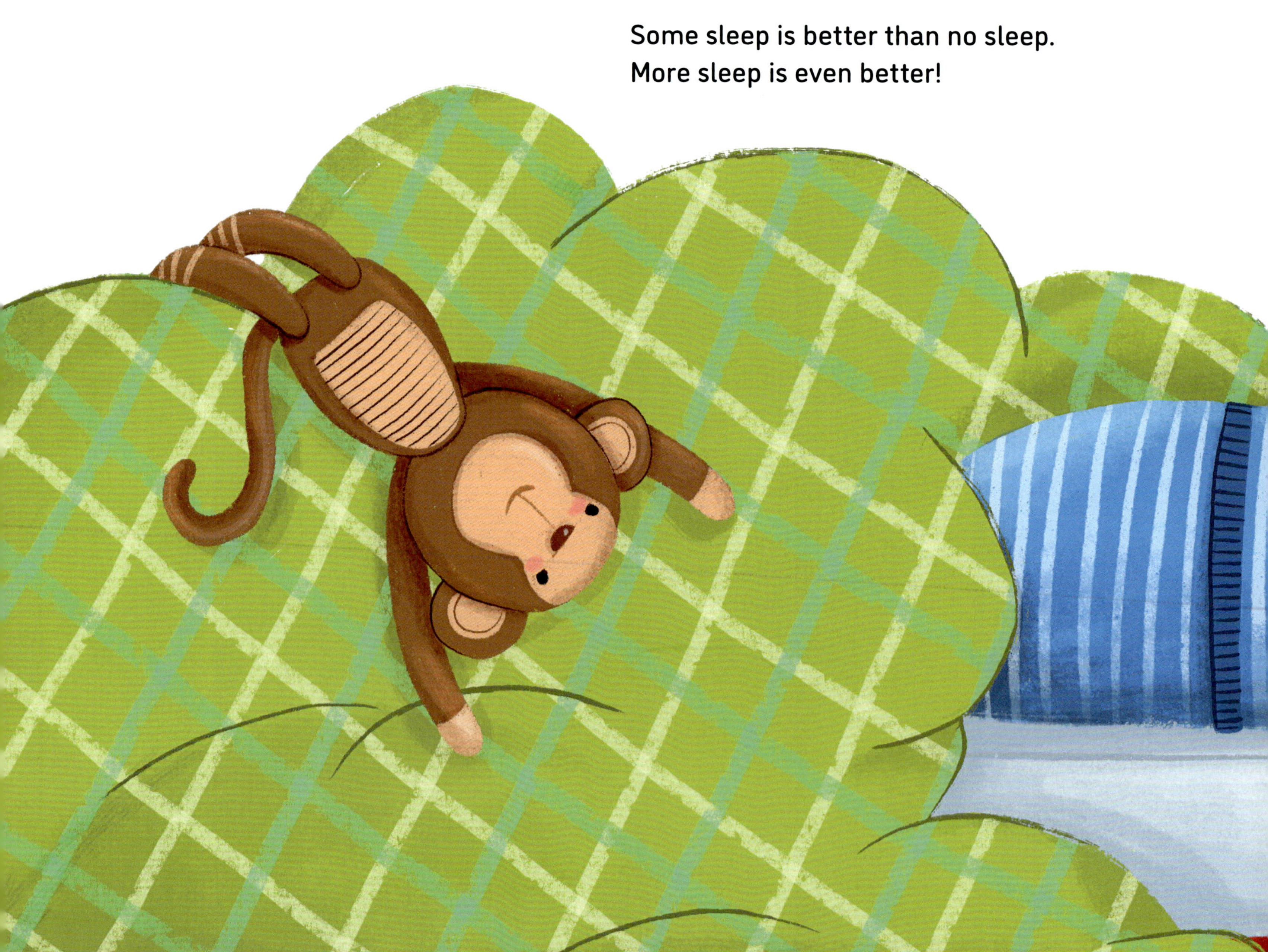

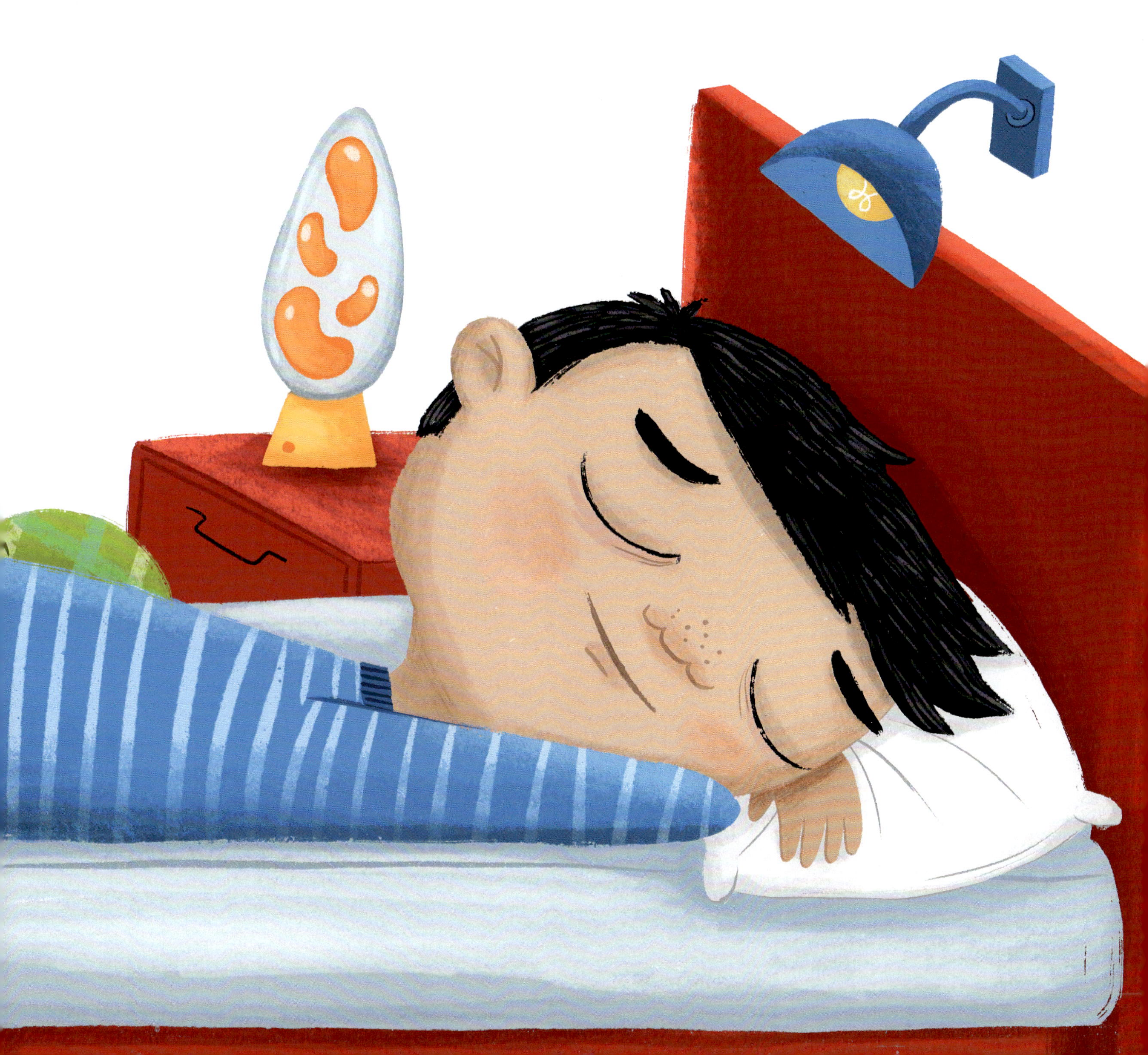

You get comfy in your bed. As you drift off to sleep, you wonder why your parents are still up. Why don't adults go to bed early like kids do?

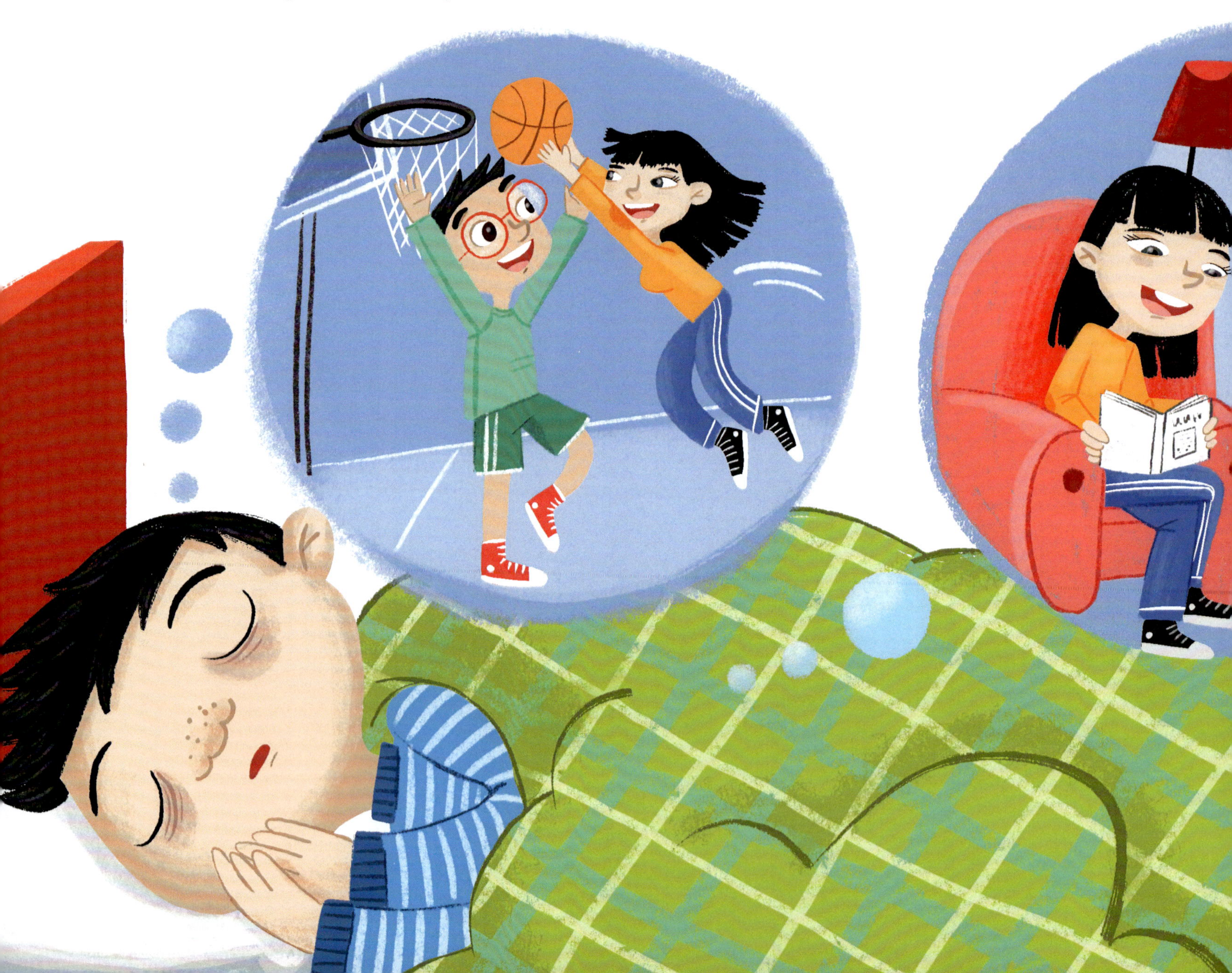

Your body knows that as a kid, you need more sleep than adults. You are still growing and your body needs rest to help that happen!

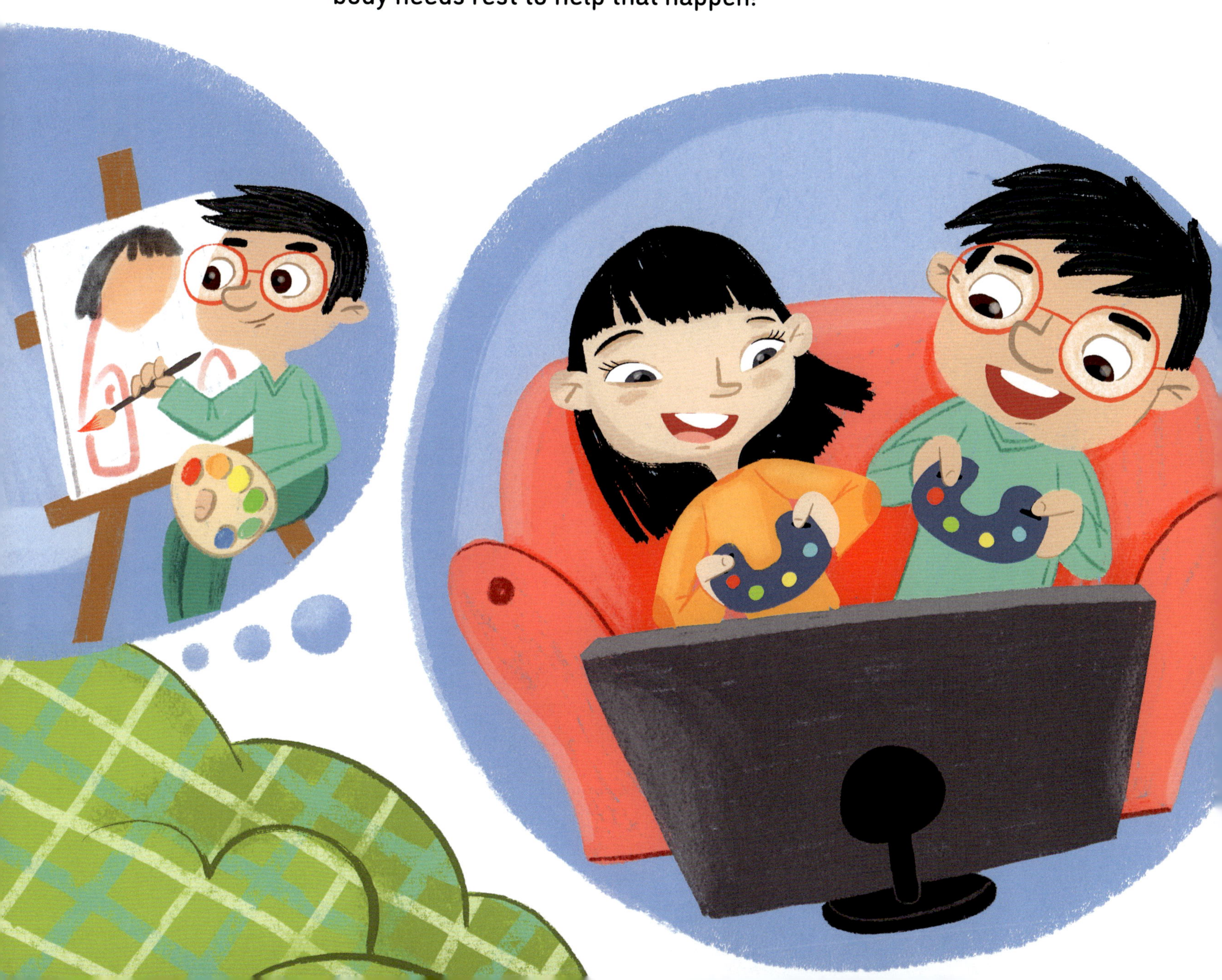

You wake up and feel great! Your brain can think straight and your body has energy. After a good night's sleep, you are ready to smack baseballs. Your body and mind are healthy again!

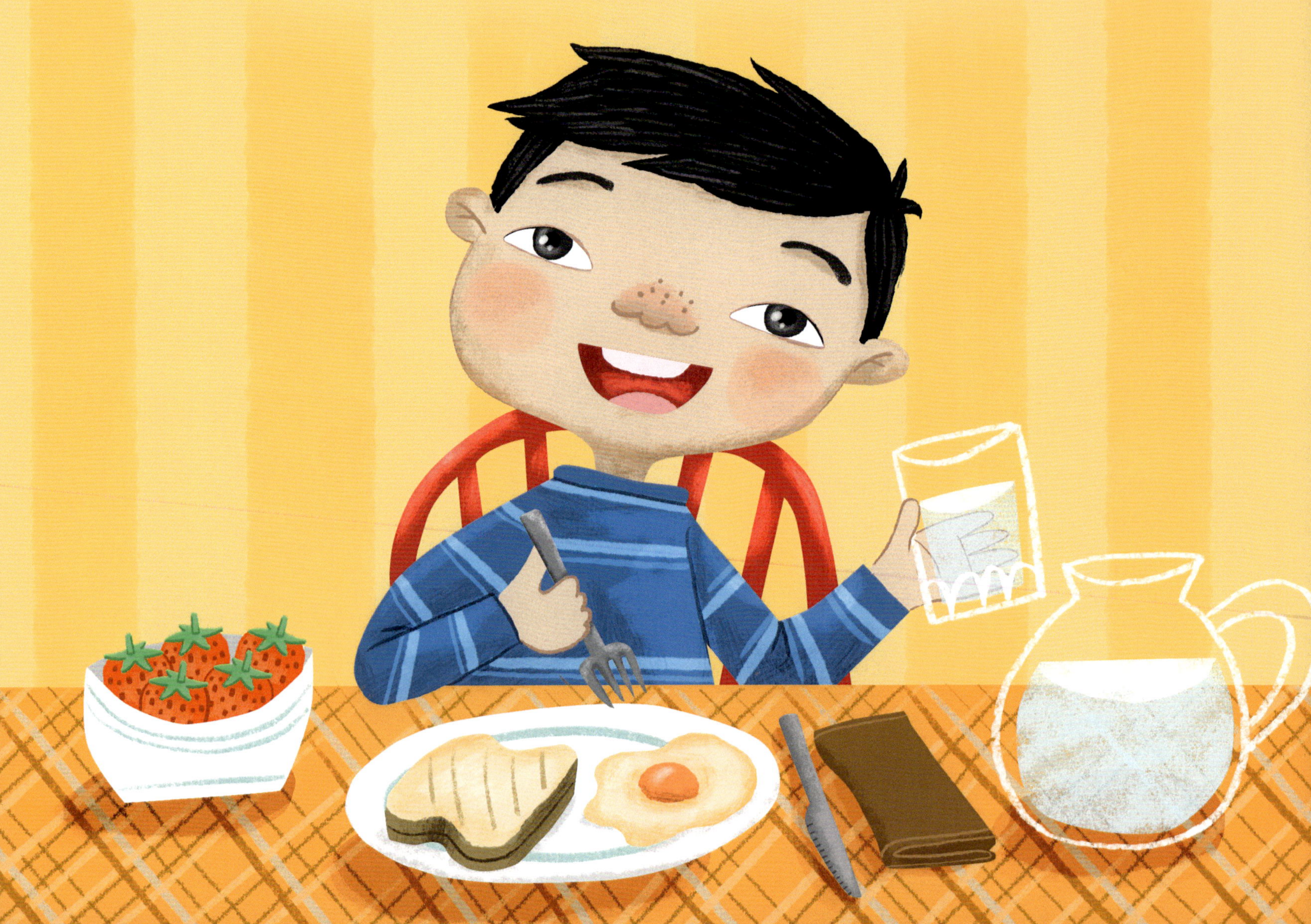

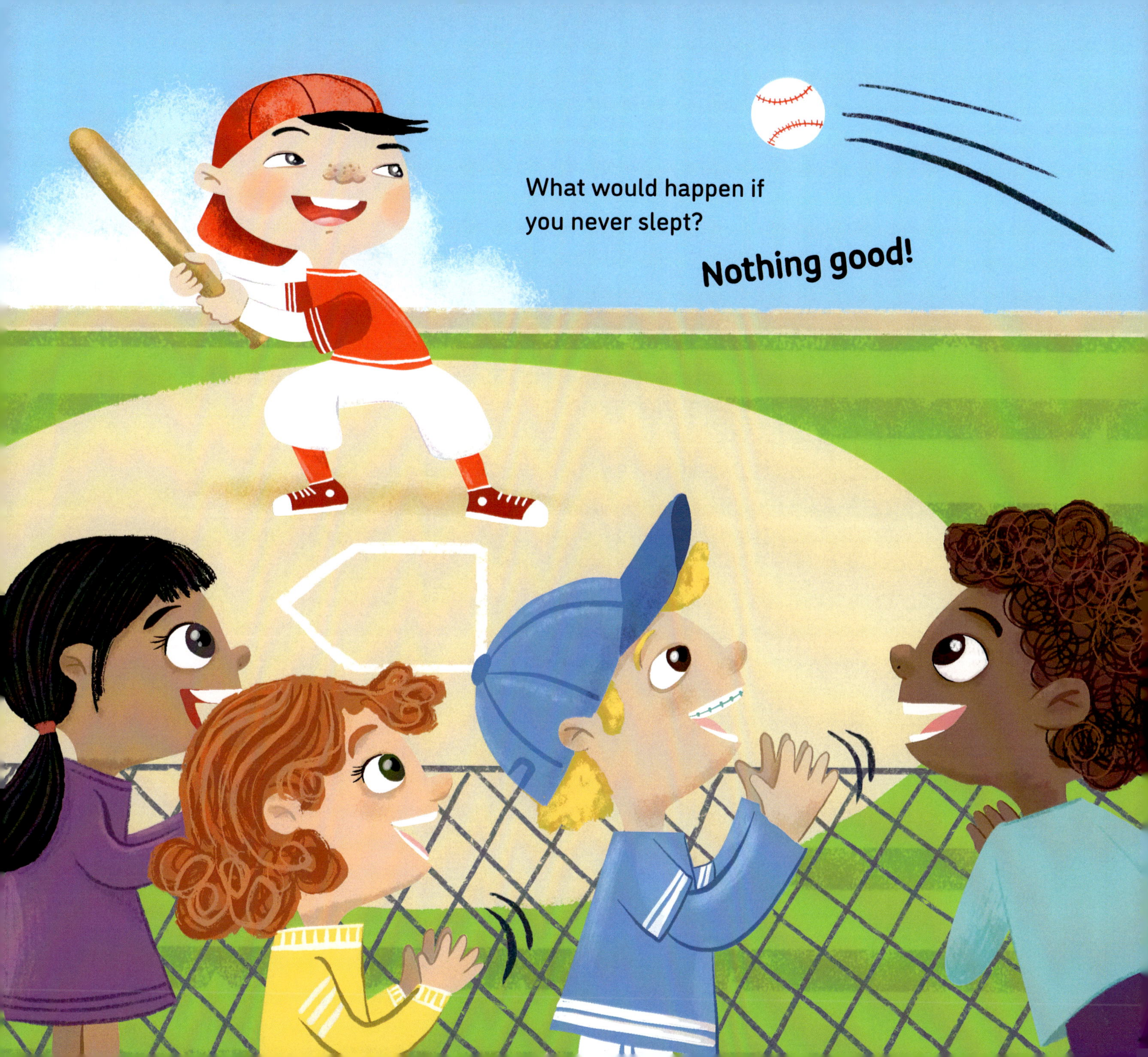

What would happen if
you never slept?

Nothing good!

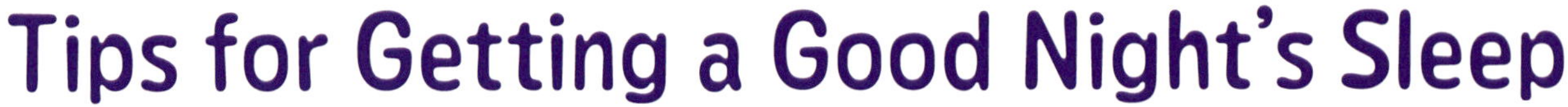

Tips for Getting a Good Night's Sleep

1. **Get plenty of exercise during the day.** This will help your body DEMAND some sleep at night!
2. **Try to keep a regular sleep schedule.** Your body will get used to going to bed and waking up around the same time!
3. **Relax before bedtime.** Do something calm and relaxing, like reading a book or writing in a journal.
4. **Avoid screens (cell phones, tablets, TV) before bed.** The blue light these devices display make it tricky to fall asleep quickly.

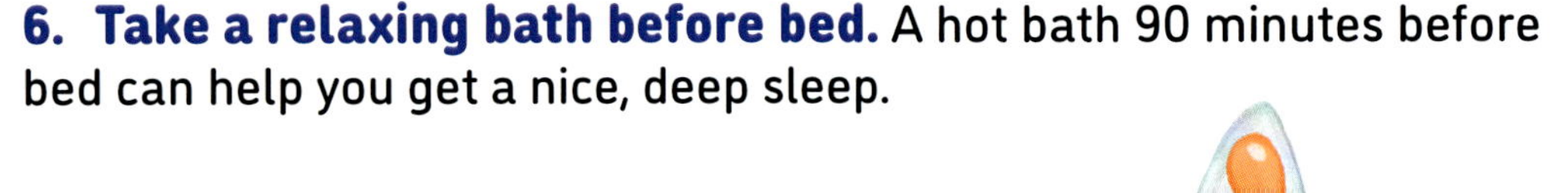

5. **A darker room is better for good sleep.** Night lights and other lights will delay the release of melatonin in your body. Melatonin is a hormone in your body that helps you fall asleep.
6. **Take a relaxing bath before bed.** A hot bath 90 minutes before bed can help you get a nice, deep sleep.

Fun Facts

WHAT?!?

You forget most of your dreams 10 minutes after waking up. Some people never remember any of their dreams.

NO KIDDING?

Getting more sleep will improve a person's memory.

REALLY?

Athletes need more sleep than most people. Sleep helps their muscles repair and restores the body's energy.

WHAT?!?

People who get good sleep live longer!

IT'S TRUE!

The brain needs sleep to function. If you actually never slept, your body would begin to shut down. You won't be able to concentrate, and you'll have trouble talking and remembering things. Get to bed!

IT'S TRUE!

A giraffe only needs 1.9 hours of sleep per day.

Glossary

confused—Uncertain or puzzled.

droopy—Hanging down or sagging.

exhausted—Very tired.

forgetful—Having a hard time remembering things.

hallucination—Something you see that is not really there.

immune system—The body's defense against sickness, infection, and disease.

Read More

Chang, Kirsten. *Getting Sleep.* Minneapolis: Bellwether Media, 2022.

Furstinger, Nancy. *How Do Dolphins Sleep?* North Mankato, Minn.: Capstone Press, 2019.

Simmons, Steven J. *Where Do Creatures Sleep at Night?* Watertown, Mass.: Charlesbridge, 2021.

Websites

Sleep for Kids: Games from the National Sleep Foundation
http://www.sleepforkids.org/html/games.html

Time for Bed?
https://kidshealth.org/en/kids/bed-game.html

What Sleep Is and Why All Kids Need It
https://kidshealth.org/en/kids/not-tired.html